POWERFUL TRANSFORMATION
THROUGH INTENTION-SETTING & SELF-INQUIRY

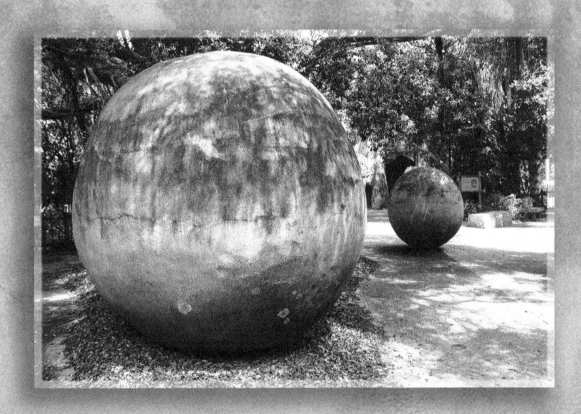

An Invitation to Self-Discovery

Marie T. Rogers, PhD

Balboa Press books may be ordered through booksellers or by contacting:

Balboa Press
A Division of Hay House
1663 Liberty Drive
Bloomington, IN 47403
www.balboapress.com
844-682-1282

Because of the dynamic nature of the Internet, any web addresses or links contained in this book may have changed since publication and may no longer be valid. The views expressed in this work are solely those of the author and do not necessarily reflect the views of the publisher, and the publisher hereby disclaims any responsibility for them.

Any people depicted in stock imagery provided by Getty Images are models, and such images are being used for illustrative purposes only.
Certain stock imagery © Getty Images.

Interior Image Credit: Paul Rogers

ISBN: 978-1-9822-5474-2 (sc)
ISBN: 978-1-9822-5475-9 (e)

Library of Congress Control Number: 2020917190

Print information available on the last page.

Balboa Press rev. date: 09/30/2020

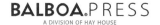

Contents

The Power of Self-Inquiry

Self-Inquiry awakens awareness that leads to true transformation.
To grow, be self-curious.
To connect, be other-curious.

My inspiration for this journal came from a decades-long journey involving two practices that together have led for profound change and healing in my life and in the lives of countless others. I am passionate about both and the time has never been more perfect than now to merge both worlds. These two worlds are **Psychology & Yoga.**

I am excited to share my knowledge and experience with you.

Psychology & Yoga

As a therapist, asking the <u>right question</u> is crucial. The right question allows for clarity, targeted problem-solving, and resolution. My training to become a psychologist emphasized brain function and behavior, and identifying patterns (emotional and behavioral) that promote or demote mental health.

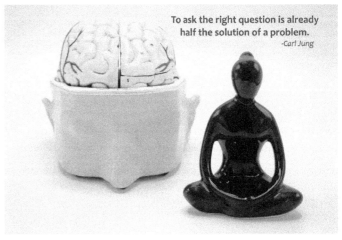

To ask the right question is already half the solution of a problem.
-Carl Jung

As a yoga practitioner and registered yoga teacher, I am intrigued by the centuries-old eastern philosophy that involves much more than exercising and stretching; although both are great for the body and brain. Yoga, derived from the Sanskrit root Yui means to join, yoke or unite. It includes breath control, body postures, and meditation, which is well outlined in Patanjali's yoga sutras and eight-fold or eight-limb path. In my yoga teacher training, I immediately became intrigued by its 7th limb – Dhyana. Dhyana refers to meditation; an internal sense of profound focus. It comes from the Sanskrit root dhyai, which means *to think of*. The combination of the two was the inspiration for the **Powerful Transformation through Intention Setting & Self-Inquiry** program.

The questions offered in your journal have been carefully chosen and sequenced to maximize the effects of self-inquiry. It is advised that you refrain from jumping ahead and answering self-inquiry questions out of order. This journal is intended to be a daily, 10-week practice. Moving at a slower pace is perfectly OK! Speeding ahead is not advised.

There is a popular Aesop's Fable titled the Tortoise and the Hare depicting a race toward a finish line between a speedy Hare and a slow-moving Tortoise. In this delightful children's story, the Tortoise, frustrated at the hare's constant belittling and disparaging remarks, initiates the challenge. Although the Tortoise is aware the hare is a formidable opponent with the gift of speed, the Tortoise nonetheless moves forward with the race, relying on a steady, unwavering focus toward a goal. To the Hare's surprise and embarrassment, the Tortoise won. The Hare had all the benefits and was favored to win (by a long-shot) but due to a sense of <u>over</u>-confidence, which led to <u>distracted</u> behaviors,

the Tortoise, with a **steady rhythm**, won the race.

This fable is applicable to so many areas in our lives and oftentimes we miss that the slow path toward a goal is favorable to the fast path leading nowhere.

The Power of Goal Setting

Setting goals helps motivate and move us forward in an onward and upward direction. Goal setting helps us organize our time, plan our day, and galvanize our resources to maximize our lives.

Goal setting provides a short- and long-term vision for what we want, and sometimes more importantly, what we do not want!

If it's not part of your vision for your life, ask yourself why you're doing it. **Clarity** and **focus** will deliver more results, life satisfaction, and peace. Ultimately, aren't these what we want for our lives and the lives of those we love?

As imperfect humans, sometimes a small bump in the road is all it takes to take us off-course. We find ourselves doing well, following an amazing plan, checking off each and every successful day, and then something happens….. an increased work demand, common cold, small emergency….. and EVERYTHING gets derailed! It is sometimes the smallest of interruptions that create the most havoc. Small interruptions are goal disruptors. And so is success. Yes, success.

We'll get to that in a minute.

The faster you get back on track after deviating off-track, the better your chances for long-term success. When you realize you missed your exit on the highway; you turn around.

You don't keep driving further and further away berating yourself for the missed exit. This applies to your everyday life. You get off-track, you immediately re-route. You will soon arrive at your destination. Be mindful of the chatter within you when things go awry. Be mindful of your thoughts. Program your internal voice for success and problem solving. Galvanize your executive functioning skills. These are the skills our frontal lobes manage and they include initiating activities and projects, organizing, planning, and completing that which was started. Think of an airplane.

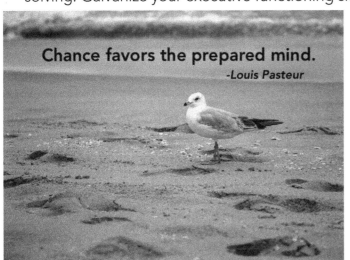

Chance favors the prepared mind.
-Louis Pasteur

There's a flight plan; a take-off, a steady on-course period of time in the air, and a landing.

Now, back to success: In order to achieve a goal, there is typically a regimen of discipline and consistency. When we reach the desired outcome, some people experience a sense of over-confidence and with reckless abandon, do away with the mindset, habits, and discipline that was needed to ensure success. Think of the hare in Aesop's fable. This is a form of self-sabotage. If you are prone to acts of self-sabotage, you are not alone! In fact, you have plenty of company. To further the discussion of self-sabotage, let's jump right into addictions.

Addictions include any behavior(s) that is/are consuming you, that you have little to no control over, and that you are trying to or need to change in order to have a better life. It's not just alcohol and drugs. It can apply to any area in your life that is or feels **out of balance**.

The proverb- **A chain is only as strong as its weakest link-** is relevant to the discussion of addictions.

The best-laid plans can easily be derailed by defaulting to patterns rooted in self-dysregulation and disconnection. We each have areas of vulnerability.← Re-read this!

These vulnerabilities become most pronounced when we are stressed. While addictive behaviors allow us to temporarily disengage and help push the pause button on what feels like insurmountable stress, it unfortunately comes with a large cost, that grows exponentially if left unchecked. There are healthy ways to push the pause or re-set button, as presented in research from the field of positive psychology by Mihaly Csikszentmihalyi, known as entering the flow state or as it is more commonly known - *entering* or *being in the zone.*

This occurs when an individual is fully immersed in an activity in which focus, creativity, and engagement are heightened. When exiting the zone, one feels a sense of fulfillment, accomplishment, and/or calm. Addictive behaviors, whether to a substance, food, exercise, work, or negative thought patterns produce different outcomes; typically, feelings of exhaustion, self-deprecation and fatigue. Mindfully targeting areas of vulnerability and addictions will yield extraordinary results in the attainment of balance and equanimity.

> **Insight, Mindfulness, & Problem Solving**
> **Knowing & Respecting Thyself!**

Each one of us has the power, at any given moment, to access a higher, more productive and calming thought, keeping in the forefront of our minds that calm is in fact a super power.

The Power of Setting an Intention

Once your goals have been established (as you journey through this program), the next step will be to galvanize the accomplishment and attainment of your goals by daily setting purposeful intentions.

Goal Setting is powerful.
Intention setting adds depth to goal setting.
It is a powerful tool in your power tool box.

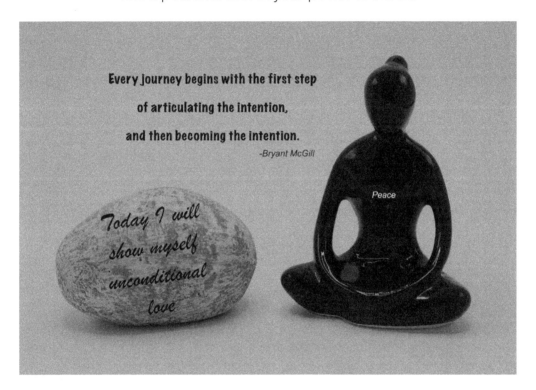

Every journey begins with the first step

of articulating the intention,

and then becoming the intention.

-Bryant McGill

Today I will show myself unconditional love

Peace

Think of intention setting as moving the ball down the field.

My Intentions		How To:
	My choices will reflect this.	1. Create a ritual around it; such as every morning.
	My thoughts will reflect this.	2. Always state intention in the positive, and never in the negative.
	My actions will reflect this.	3. Connect the intention with a goal, or with your goals (as a whole).

Our thoughts control the flow of energy within and they can quickly and strongly become habitual. Unfortunately, we tend to regurgitate the same thoughts over and over.

This stifles creativity.
It also stifles growth, and motivation, and energy.
Many of us are fatigued from the heaviness of our thoughts
and the 'stuckness' of our feelings.

We need space for new and better
thoughts to germinate.
This will increase energy.
Energy is our life-line.

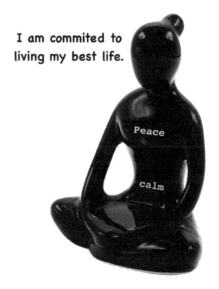

I am commited to
living my best life.

Peace

calm

The Power of Gratitude

There is no dearth of psychological research documenting the therapeutic value of expressing gratitude. In fact, its benefits are often and easily overlooked.

If we do practice gratitude, it is often once per year, perhaps at Thanksgiving, or when things are going "really well."

It is encouraged that you integrate a gratitude practice into your life more frequently.

Daily is an optimal prescription!

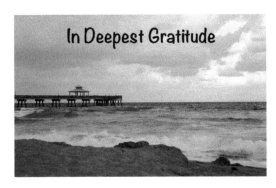

Here are just a few benefits:
- Improves physical health
- Improves mental health
- Improves confidence
- Improves immune function
- Improves sleep
- Improves relationships
- Improves resiliency

Special bonus: The frequent expression of gratitude has been known to increase the likelihood of manifesting opportunities. Grateful people seem to be magnets for good luck!

Let's take the power of gratitude one step further→ showing it to others.

The power of showing appreciation cannot be understated. It has the power to strengthen relationships, while its absence generally destroys them.

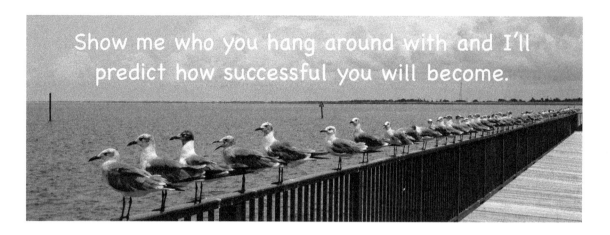
Show me who you hang around with and I'll predict how successful you will become.

The Power of My Sphere of Influence

Humans are hard-wired for connection. This includes introverts, extraverts, and ambiverts.

Our need for connection means we are more influenced by others' behaviors and actions than we may wish to acknowledge.

If you want to see where you're headed, take inventory of who you're hanging out with as these are the people who have the greatest influence on you, your choices, behaviors, thoughts and feelings. We often do not like to acknowledge this; however, the growing field of neuro- and behavioral science supports this observation.

Without getting too sciency, research supports the influence others have on us and this evidence is, at least, partially based on mirror neurons. Mirror neurons are neurons in our brain that fire when we do something or when we observe someone else doing the same thing. These neurons allow us to adapt to another's point of view and almost inadvertently and subconsciously take on others' characteristics and habits.

Mirror neurons permit us to deepen shared human experiences.

> **You are the average of the 5 people you spend the most time with.**
> **Jim Rohn**

Know thy network.
Know thyself.
Heal thyself.

The Power of Journaling

Capture your story in writing

Research has well documented that journaling and self-reflection are powerful agents of change, insight, healing, and growth.

Whether journaling for life management, creative expression, problem solving or just to record your history, the act of taking pen to paper and writing is powerful.

When we write, as opposed to typing or just *thinking about*, a unique neural circuitry is activated. This automatic activation often leads to deeper thinking and processing. It often leads to *connecting the dots*.
When we connect the dots, we see patterns.
Patterns connect us to insight!

We learn by writing!

Journaling, a solitary activity, also engages mindfulness.

Mindfulness leads to clarity, calmness and creativity.

Through Mindfulness, we will access higher thinking.
We will be able to see **(c)** more clearly; see **(c)** the bigger picture; see **(c)** the solutions.
By flipping the **(c)** in rea<u>c</u>tivity to the front of the line (or word), we get **c**reativity.

A <u>creative</u> life is much better than a <u>reactive</u> life!

Through the conscientious and intentional process of connecting ourselves
to our pen and journal, we connect more deeply inwardly.
This connection is often experienced as an expression of self-love.
By doing this, we are giving ourselves the gift of time; time
to be with ourselves to reflect, feel and think.

Our frontal lobes, responsible for <u>executive functioning</u>, thrive when journaling.

The question: **"What is my next action step?"** when journaled promotes critical thinking and focus that is unmatched by almost any other activity.

Journaling connects left and right brain hemispheres.
Journaling connects our rational and our intuitive self.

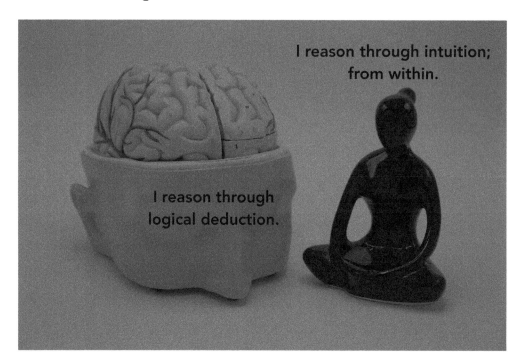

The Power of Creating a Daily Morning Ritual

Bringing It All Together

One of my all-time favorite sayings or actually theories comes from Canadian psychologist, Donald O. Hebb and it is known as the <u>Hebbian theory</u>:

Neurons that fire together, wire together.

What does this mean and how is it applicable?

Our brain cells communicate. Remember the mirror neurons? Our brains communicate through neurotransmitters. One cell sends a message; the other cell receives it.

This beautiful communication system is known as *neuronal firing.*

When there is frequent communication, the connection strengthens.
The stronger the connection, the faster it becomes.
It then becomes so automatic that we no longer have to give much thought to this action.
Just like that, a **habit** is formed!

This can be desirable if the paired association is productive. For example, I wake up in the morning and immediately work out. No questions asked. It's just what I do!

However, this may not be a good thing if my habit involves waking up and erratically and hurriedly grabbing a sugary pastry, racing to get to work, immediately checking my e-mail (before grounding myself to my day), and responding to everyone else's demands and requests. Before 9am, fatigue and exhaustion have already settled in.

We can all see how and where this day is going to go.

I wish this were the exception. It's not. It's the norm for so many of us.

We've habituated to becoming Human Doers, and not Human Beings.

When Do comes before Be
A recipe for burn-out.

When Be comes before Do,
We feel inspired, motivated, and energized.

When consciously applying the Hebbian principle, we can, over time, establish strong and powerful neuronal wiring leading to great habits that will last a lifetime.

If **practice makes perfect**, then let's in full awareness decide
exactly which practice we want to make perfect!

The next step is to connect the Hebbian Theory with the Morning Ritual.

The morning ritual, practiced by countless successful people around our planet, will help
us live with intention, with integrity, and with alignment of who we are and meant to be.
It connects us with our soul, our passion, our purpose
and with the highest version of ourselves!

Starting your day with setting your intention, after thoughtfully identifying and
reflecting on your goals, will do more for your mental and physical health than almost
any other single activity. Whether you are an experienced intention-setter and journal
enthusiast or whether the concept of setting an intention and writing in a journal is
foreign to you, this 10-week program is a great addition to or a starting point to the
achievement of **Sophrosyne,** an ancient Greek concept of excellence and integrity,
promoting

Soundness of Mind
Self-Control
Self-Knowledge

Just as there will be experienced intention-setters and journalers and
novice intention-setters and journalers, there will also be individual
differences in where we each are on the path to healing.

It is important to respect our boundaries, vulnerabilities and triggers. What can feel
like a fun path to furthering one's self-awareness to someone who is currently in a
good place emotionally can be experienced as triggering and upsetting to another
who may not be in such a comfortable place; emotionally and/or physically.
Our journeys and our healing are our responsibilities and unique to our circumstances.
It's important to not compare our life with that of anybody else's.
We, each, have a unique path.
However, we were not meant to walk it alone.
We were made for connection.

While this daily practice is solitary, meaning you are alone with your thoughts and journal,
and it is intended to invite you to think, feel, and process,
and to evoke a full range of emotions,
it was not intended for you to necessarily keep your insights and discoveries to yourself.

If alone and keeping to yourself are your preferences and you're OK, then continue.

However, you may wish to share this experience with others.
Trusted others.

This can be your therapist, life coach, best friend, spiritual leader, etc. Processing the questions with a trusted individual or cohesive group can bring upon profound effects and healing. Whereas the rise of emotions is normal and to be expected, feeling stuck and/or overwhelmed may require consulting with a licensed psychotherapist, if you are not already seeing one. Do not hesitate to reach out for support.

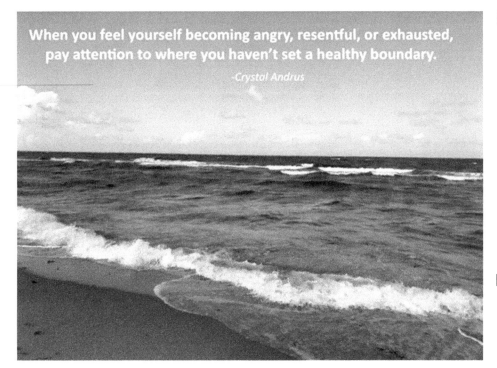

When you feel yourself becoming angry, resentful, or exhausted, pay attention to where you haven't set a healthy boundary.

-Crystal Andrus

Respecting ourselves is a true act of self-love.

Respecting our boundaries helps us grow.

When we respect our own boundaries, we gain self-trust.

Self-trust helps us establish healthy boundaries with others.

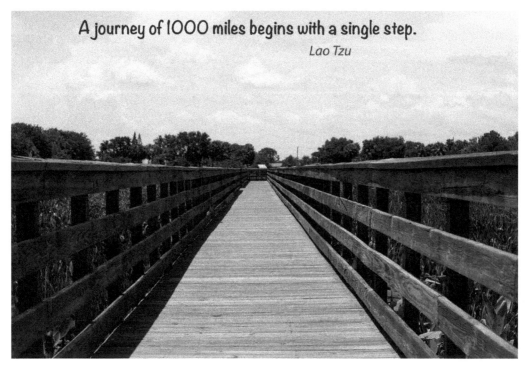

A journey of 1000 miles begins with a single step.
Lao Tzu

May each of your steps lead you down this path!

Step 1: Identify your goals; short & long range, and sphere of influence.

Step 2: Carve out time each morning to set your intention for the day. This should take seconds to maybe, several minutes. You are also invited to reflect on and write 3 things you're grateful for and to connect your day to a goal. Always consider the most powerful thought you have access to as you visualize your day.

Step 3: On the second day in a week's cycle, you will be invited to reflect upon a Self-Inquiry question. <u>This is your question for the week</u>. Give each question the attention it deserves and time. Reflect on this question at different points in your week allowing for at least one of the deep reflections to occur when in an "alpha brain wave" state. This occurs when daydreaming or deeply relaxed. Meditation, praying, mindfulness, and exercise, especially yoga, help access this state. We also enter this state before falling asleep.

Step 4: On the seventh day, you will have the opportunity to reflect on your week and plan the week ahead. As with the self-inquiry questions, allow yourself time to reflect on your week. Grab your favorite beverage and pen, find a calm location, diffuse a healing aromatherapy essential oil, and mindfully connect with yourself. Extra tip: I have created my personal music and sound therapy playlist to play in the background when journaling. You may want to do this as well.

REPEAT and know that you are on the path. You are exactly where you need to be. All that you have been through is preparing you for the present moment and who you are growing into. **Grow**

It is by growing and through personal development that we are able to bring our best energy to others and to our circumstances.

My GOALs

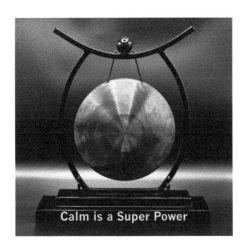

Calm is a Super Power

Establishing:

- My 30-Day GOALs
- My 90-Day GOALs
- My 1-Year GOALs
- My 5-Year GOALs

Plan it. Do it.

My Personal Goals for the next 30 days: **Date in 30 days:** ___/_____/_____
1. _____
2. _____
3. _____

My Personal Goals for the next 90 days: **Date in 90 days:** ___/_____/_____
1. _____
2. _____
3. _____

My Personal Goals for the next year: **Date in 1 year:** ___/_____/_____
1. _____
2. _____
3. _____

My Personal Goals for the next 5 years: **Date in 5 years:** ___/_____/_____
1. _____
2. _____
3. _____

My sphere of influence involves the 5 people with whom I spend the most time.
They include:
1. _____
2. _____
3. _____
4. _____
5. _____

Week 1

Day 1   Date: _____

Today's Intention:

_____
_____
_____
_____

Today I am grateful for:

- _____
- _____
- _____

Which goal will I focus on today? _____

Day 2   Date: _____

Today's Intention:

_____
_____
_____
_____

Today I am grateful for:

- _____
- _____
- _____

Which goal will I focus on today? _____

Go to your 1st Self-Inquiry

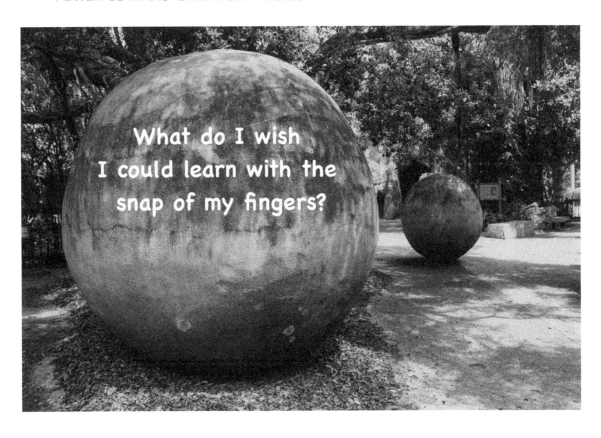

What do I wish I could learn with the snap of my fingers?

_____
_____
_____
_____

How would my life be different if I learned this? _____
_____
_____

Am I motivated to create a plan to incorporate learning this into my life right now? If yes, what is my plan? _____
_____
_____

If no, is this something I would like to learn in the future? If yes, how will I add this to my life?
_____
_____
_____

If not now, and not in the foreseeable future, ask yourself and reflect on why
you identified this as something you wish you could learn.

Day 3 Date_____

Today's Intention:

_____
_____
_____
_____

Today I am grateful for:
- _____
- _____
- _____

Which goal will I focus on today? _____

Day 4 Date: _____

Today's Intention:

_____
_____
_____
_____

Today I am grateful for:
- _____
- _____
- _____

Which goal will I focus on today? _____

Day 5 Date: _____

Today's Intention:

_____
_____
_____
_____

Today I am grateful for:

- _____
- _____
- _____

Which goal will I focus on today? _____

Day 6   Date: _____

Today's Intention:

_____
_____
_____
_____

Today I am grateful for:

- _____
- _____
- _____

Which goal will I focus on today? _____

Day 7   Date: _____

Today's Intention:

_____
_____
_____
_____

Today I am grateful for:

- _____
- _____
- _____

Which goal will I focus on today? _____

End of week 1

Go to Week 1's Let's Reflect

Week 1 is now completed. Let's reflect:

What went well? _____
_____
_____

What did not go well? _____
_____
_____
_____

Did I live in alignment with my goals? _____

If yes, what felt aligned? _____

    What can I do to strengthen this alignment in Week 2? _____
    _____

If no, what felt misaligned? _____

    What can I do differently in Week 2? _____
    _____

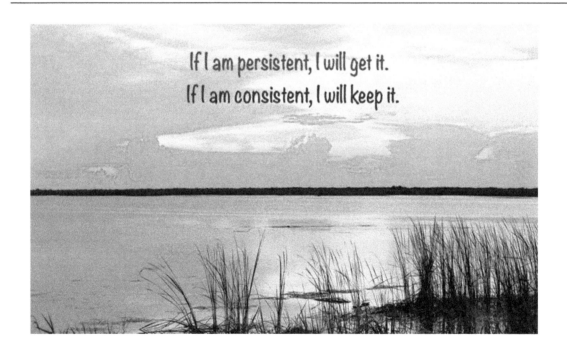

If I am persistent, I will get it.
If I am consistent, I will keep it.

Week 2

Day 1   Date: _____

Today's Intention:

_____
_____
_____
_____

Today I am grateful for:

- _____
- _____
- _____

Which goal will I focus on today? _____

Day 2   Date: _____

Today's Intention:

_____
_____
_____
_____

Today I am grateful for:

- _____
- _____
- _____

Which goal will I focus on today? _____

Go to your 2nd Self-Inquiry

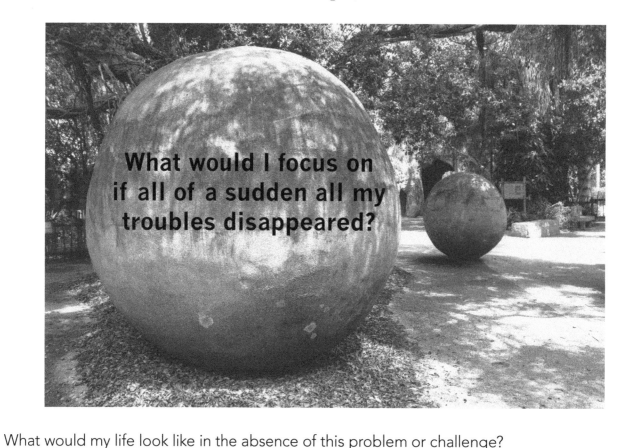

What would my life look like in the absence of this problem or challenge?

_____
_____
_____
_____
_____
_____
_____
_____
_____
_____
_____
_____
_____
_____
_____
_____
_____
_____
_____

Day 3   Date_____

Today's Intention:

_____
_____
_____
_____

Today I am grateful for:

- _____
- _____
- _____

Which goal will I focus on today? _____

Day 4   Date: _____

Today's Intention:

_____
_____
_____
_____

Today I am grateful for:

- _____
- _____
- _____

Which goal will I focus on today? _____

Day 5   Date: _____

Today's Intention:

_____
_____
_____
_____

Today I am grateful for:

- _____
- _____
- _____

Which goal will I focus on today? _____

Day 6   Date: _____

Today's Intention:

_____
_____
_____
_____

Today I am grateful for:

- _____
- _____
- _____

Which goal will I focus on today? _____

Day 7   Date: _____

Today's Intention:

_____
_____
_____
_____

Today I am grateful for:

- _____
- _____
- _____

Which goal will I focus on today? _____

Go to Week 2's Let's Reflect

Week 2 is now completed. Let's reflect:

What went well? _____
_____
_____

What did not go well? _____
_____
_____

Did I live in alignment with my goals? _____
_____
_____

If yes, what felt aligned? _____
    What can I do to strengthen this alignment in Week 3? _____
_____
_____

If no, what felt misaligned? _____
    What can I do differently in Week 3? _____
_____
_____

Answers easily flow to me

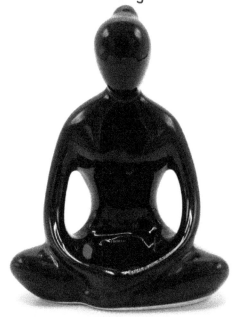

Week 3

Day 1   Date: _____

Today's Intention:

_____
_____
_____
_____

Today I am grateful for:

- _____
- _____
- _____

Which goal will I focus on today? _____

Day 2   Date: _____

Today's Intention:

_____
_____
_____
_____

Today I am grateful for:

- _____
- _____
- _____

Which goal will I focus on today? _____

Go to your 3rd Self-Inquiry

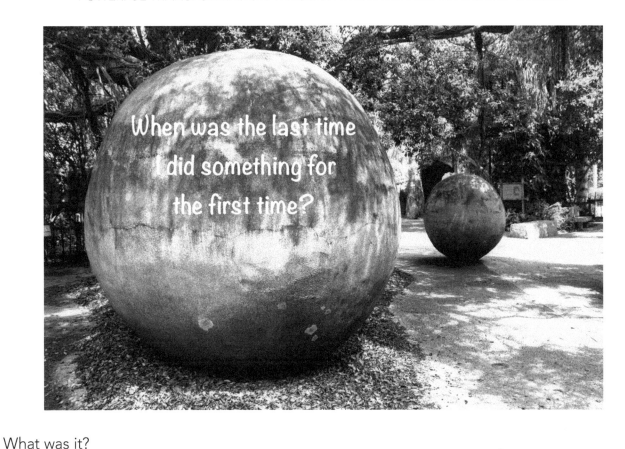

What was it?
How did it feel to try or do something new?
What led you to this experience?

_____
_____
_____
_____
_____
_____
_____
_____
_____
_____
_____
_____
_____
_____

The power behind this question is to assess whether or not you're living the same life day-in- and-day-out or whether there is enough variety and growth to keep things stimulating. Routine is good. Consistency helps in goal setting. However, too much routine and adherence to consistency can create a dull life.

Day 3   Date_____

Today's Intention:

_____
_____
_____
_____

Today I am grateful for:
- _____
- _____
- _____

Which goal will I focus on today? _____

Day 4   Date: _____

Today's Intention:

_____
_____
_____
_____

Today I am grateful for:
- _____
- _____
- _____

Which goal will I focus on today? _____

Day 5   Date: _____

Today's Intention:

_____
_____
_____
_____

Today I am grateful for:

- _____
- _____
- _____

Which goal will I focus on today? _____

Day 6   Date: _____

Today's Intention:

_____
_____
_____
_____

Today I am grateful for:

- _____
- _____
- _____

Which goal will I focus on today? _____

Day 7   Date: _____

Today's Intention:

_____
_____
_____
_____

Today I am grateful for:

- _____
- _____
- _____

Which goal will I focus on today? _____

Go to Week 3's Let's Reflect

Week 3 is now completed. Let's reflect:

What went well? _____
_____
_____

What did not go well? _____
_____
_____

Did I live in alignment with my goals? _____
_____
_____

If yes, what felt aligned? _____
    What can I do to strengthen this alignment in Week 4? _____
_____
_____

If no, what felt misaligned? _____
    What can I do differently in Week 4? _____
_____
_____

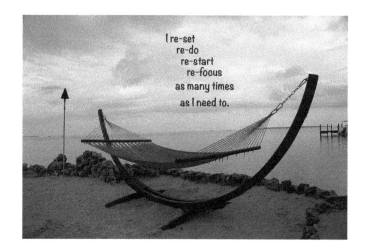

Week 4

Day 1   Date: _____

Today's Intention:

_____
_____
_____
_____

Today I am grateful for:

- _____
- _____
- _____

Which goal will I focus on today? _____

Day 2   Date: _____

Today's Intention:

_____
_____
_____
_____

Today I am grateful for:

- _____
- _____
- _____

Which goal will I focus on today? _____

Go to your 4th Self-Inquiry

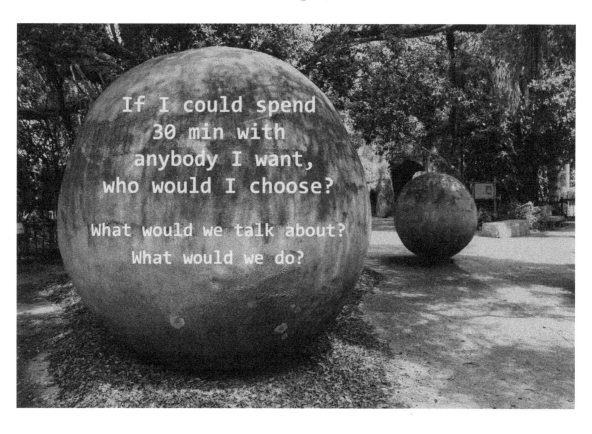

If I could spend
30 min with
anybody I want,
who would I choose?

What would we talk about?
What would we do?

Day 3   Date_____

Today's Intention:

_____
_____
_____
_____

Today I am grateful for:

- _____
- _____
- _____

Which goal will I focus on today? _____

Day 4   Date: _____

Today's Intention:

_____
_____
_____
_____

Today I am grateful for:

- _____
- _____
- _____

Which goal will I focus on today? _____

Day 5   Date: _____

Today's Intention:

_____
_____
_____
_____

Today I am grateful for:

- _____
- _____
- _____

Which goal will I focus on today? _____

Day 6   Date: _____

Today's Intention:

_____
_____
_____
_____

Today I am grateful for:

- _____
- _____
- _____

Which goal will I focus on today? _____

Day 7   Date: _____

Today's Intention:

_____
_____
_____
_____

Today I am grateful for:

- _____
- _____
- _____

Which goal will I focus on today? _____

Go to Week 4's Let's Reflect

Week 4 is now completed. Let's reflect:

What went well? _____

_____

_____

What did not go well? _____

_____

_____

Did I live in alignment with my goals? _____

_____

_____

If yes, what felt aligned? _____

What can I do to strengthen this alignment in Week 5? _____

_____

_____

If no, what felt misaligned? _____

What can I do differently in Week 5? _____

_____

_____

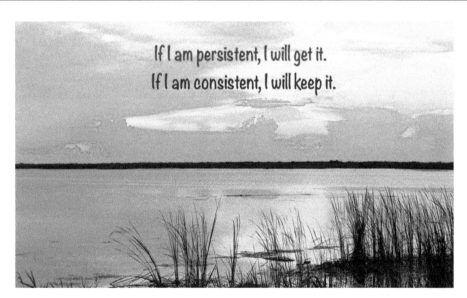

If I am persistent, I will get it.
If I am consistent, I will keep it.

It is now a month later. New behaviors typically take approximately one month to develop into new habits. Remember the Hebbian principle:

Neurons that fire together, wire together.

It's been a month, I am now engaging in the following positive habits: _____

_____

_____

_____

_____

_____

_____

_____

My life, My Choices:

- Revisit your goals.
- Revise as needed. Sometimes as we grow, our goals grow and as we change, our goals change.
- How is my Sphere of Influence looking? Have I changed who I spend time with? Did I need to? Do I need to?
- Remind yourself that growth is a personal and powerful choice. At any point we can change the trajectory of our lives by a simple choice.

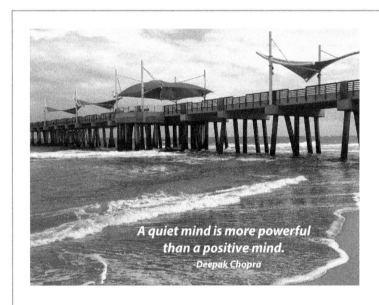

A quiet mind is more powerful than a positive mind.
-Deepak Chopra

How can I feel more empowered with each passing day?

Week 5

Day 1   Date: _____

Today's Intention:

_____
_____
_____
_____

Today I am grateful for:

- _____
- _____
- _____

Which goal will I focus on today? _____

Day 2   Date: _____

Today's Intention:

_____
_____
_____
_____

Today I am grateful for:

- _____
- _____
- _____

Which goal will I focus on today? _____

Go to your 5th Self-Inquiry

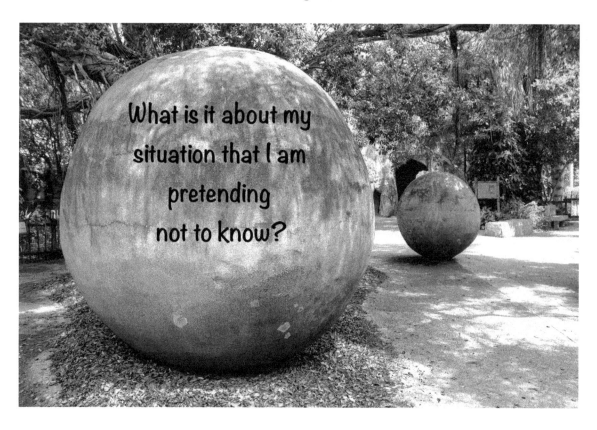

What is it about my
situation that I am
pretending
not to know?

Day 3   Date_____

Today's Intention:

_____
_____
_____
_____

Today I am grateful for:

- _____
- _____
- _____

Which goal will I focus on today? _____

Day 4   Date: _____

Today's Intention:

_____
_____
_____
_____

Today I am grateful for:

- _____
- _____
- _____

Which goal will I focus on today? _____

Day 5   Date: _____

Today's Intention:

_____
_____
_____
_____

Today I am grateful for:

- _____
- _____
- _____

Which goal will I focus on today? _____

Day 6   Date: _____

Today's Intention:

_____
_____
_____
_____

Today I am grateful for:

- _____
- _____
- _____

Which goal will I focus on today? _____

Day 7   Date: _____

Today's Intention:

_____
_____
_____
_____

Today I am grateful for:

- _____
- _____
- _____

Which goal will I focus on today? _____

Go to Week 5's Let's Reflect

Week 5 is now completed. Let's reflect:

What went well? _____
_____
_____

What did not go well? _____
_____
_____

Did I live in alignment with my goals? _____
_____
_____

If yes, what felt aligned? _____
    What can I do to strengthen this alignment in Week 6? _____
_____
_____

If no, what felt misaligned? _____
    What can I do differently in Week 6? _____
_____
_____

Answers easily flow to me

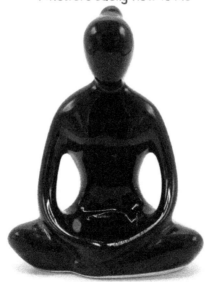

Week 6

Day 1   Date: _____

Today's Intention:

_____
_____
_____
_____

Today I am grateful for:

- _____
- _____
- _____

Which goal will I focus on today? _____

Day 2   Date: _____

Today's Intention:

_____
_____
_____
_____

Today I am grateful for:

- _____
- _____
- _____

Which goal will I focus on today? _____

Go to your 6th Self-Inquiry

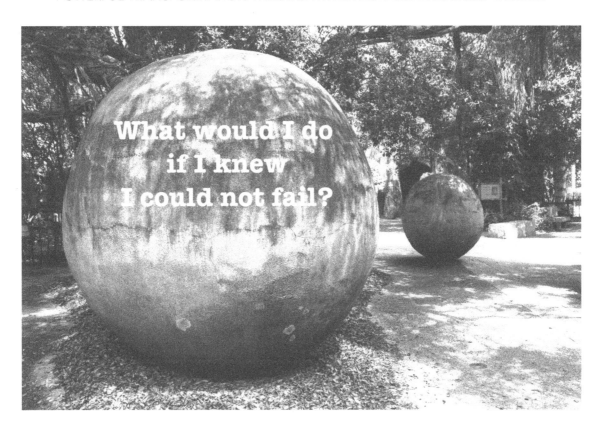

Day 3   Date_____

Today's Intention:

_____
_____
_____
_____

Today I am grateful for:

- _____
- _____
- _____

Which goal will I focus on today? _____

Day 4   Date: _____

Today's Intention:

_____
_____
_____
_____

Today I am grateful for:

- _____
- _____
- _____

Which goal will I focus on today? _____

Day 5   Date: _____

Today's Intention:

_____
_____
_____
_____

Today I am grateful for:

- _____
- _____
- _____

Which goal will I focus on today? _____

Day 6   Date: _____

Today's Intention:

_____
_____
_____
_____

Today I am grateful for:

- _____
- _____
- _____

Which goal will I focus on today? _____

Day 7   Date: _____

Today's Intention:

_____
_____
_____
_____

Today I am grateful for:

- _____
- _____
- _____

Which goal will I focus on today? _____

Go to Week 6's Let's Reflect

Week 6 is now completed. Let's reflect:

What went well? _____
_____
_____

What did not go well? _____
_____
_____

Did I live in alignment with my goals? _____
_____
_____

If yes, what felt aligned? _____
    What can I do to strengthen this alignment in Week 7? _____
    _____
    _____

If no, what felt misaligned? _____
    What can I do differently in Week 7? _____
    _____
    _____

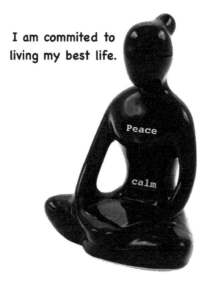

I am commited to living my best life.

Week 7

Day 1   Date: _____

Today's Intention:

_____
_____
_____
_____

Today I am grateful for:

- _____
- _____
- _____

Which goal will I focus on today? _____

Day 2   Date: _____

Today's Intention:

_____
_____
_____
_____

Today I am grateful for:

- _____
- _____
- _____

Which goal will I focus on today? _____

Go to your 7th Self-Inquiry

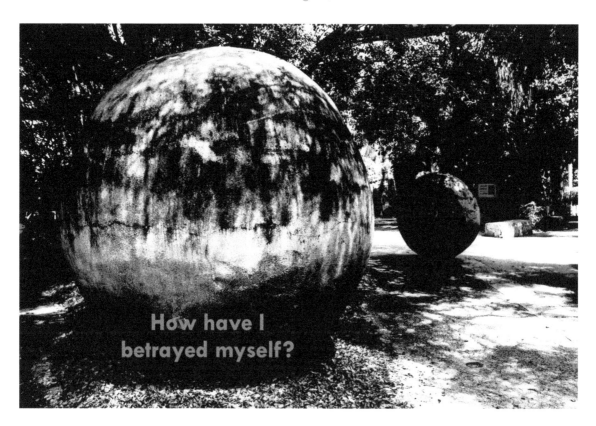

How have I
betrayed myself?

Spend some quality time with yourself to answer this question. It's deep. This is an opportunity for honest self-reflection and self-evaluation. Try not to blame yourself or others and try not to look for excuses or even explanations. Whereas rationalization can be a helpful defense or coping mechanism, we are not looking for that here. We're looking for raw, for truth, for awakening.

We're looking to unblock stuck emotions.

_____
_____
_____
_____
_____
_____
_____
_____
_____
_____
_____
_____
_____
_____

The power in this self-inquiry is to unlock areas in your life that may be blocked.

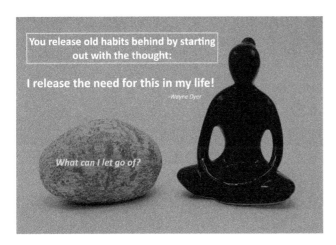

- How can I forgive myself?
- How can I forgive others, or a particular someone?
- What did I learn from this experience?
- How can I grab the lesson, use it as a growth experience, and release it?

_____
_____
_____
_____
_____
_____
_____
_____
_____
_____
_____
_____
_____
_____
_____
_____
_____

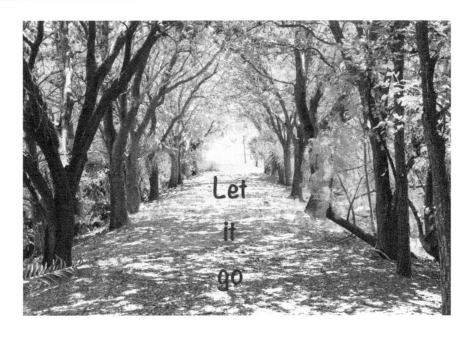

Day 3   Date_____

Today's Intention:

_____
_____
_____
_____

Today I am grateful for:
- _____
- _____
- _____

Which goal will I focus on today? _____

Day 4   Date: _____

Today's Intention:

_____
_____
_____
_____

Today I am grateful for:
- _____
- _____
- _____

Which goal will I focus on today? _____

Day 5   Date: _____

Today's Intention:

_____
_____
_____
_____

Today I am grateful for:

- _____
- _____
- _____

Which goal will I focus on today? _____

Day 6   Date: _____

Today's Intention:

_____
_____
_____
_____

Today I am grateful for:

- _____
- _____
- _____

Which goal will I focus on today? _____

Day 7   Date: _____

Today's Intention:

_____
_____
_____
_____

Today I am grateful for:

- _____
- _____
- _____

Which goal will I focus on today? _____

Go to Week 7's Let's Reflect

Week 7 is now completed. Let's reflect:

What went well? _____
_____
_____

What did not go well? _____
_____
_____

Did I live in alignment with my goals? _____
_____
_____

If yes, what felt aligned? _____
    What can I do to strengthen this alignment in Week 8? _____
_____
_____

If no, what felt misaligned? _____
    What can I do differently in Week 8? _____
_____
_____

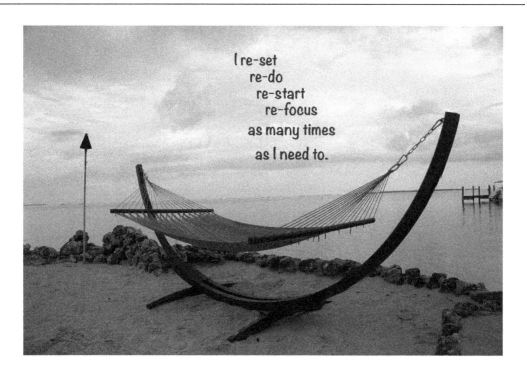

Week 8

Day 1   Date: _____

Today's Intention:

_____
_____
_____
_____

Today I am grateful for:
- _____
- _____
- _____

Which goal will I focus on today? _____

Day 2   Date: _____

Today's Intention:

_____
_____
_____
_____

Today I am grateful for:
- _____
- _____
- _____

Which goal will I focus on today? _____

Go to your 8th Self-Inquiry

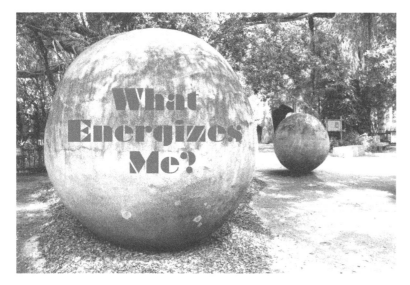

List of Personal Energizers:

1. _____
2. _____
3. _____
4. _____
5. _____
6. _____
7. _____
8. _____
9. _____

My thoughts:

_____
_____
_____
_____
_____

When in my life did I feel the MOST ENERGIZED?

_____
_____
_____
_____
_____
_____

What depletes me of my energy? _____

_____
_____
_____
_____
_____
_____

After reflecting and identifying your energizers, I invite you to take a photo of this and keep it nearby. It will be a reference that will help you when about to do something addictive, self-destructive, self-sabotaging, mindless, etc. When we're feeling weak or vulnerable, we often cannot easily reference or recall what makes us feel stronger.

Day 3   Date_____

Today's Intention:

_____
_____
_____
_____

Today I am grateful for:
- _____
- _____
- _____

Which goal will I focus on today? _____

Day 4   Date: _____

Today's Intention:

_____
_____
_____
_____

Today I am grateful for:
- _____
- _____
- _____

Which goal will I focus on today? _____

Day 5   Date: _____

Today's Intention:

_____
_____
_____
_____

Today I am grateful for:
- _____
- _____
- _____

Which goal will I focus on today? _____

Day 6   Date: _____

Today's Intention:

_____
_____
_____
_____

Today I am grateful for:
- _____
- _____
- _____

Which goal will I focus on today? _____

Day 7   Date: _____

Today's Intention:

_____
_____
_____
_____

Today I am grateful for:
- _____
- _____
- _____

Which goal will I focus on today? _____

Go to Week 8's Let's Reflect

Week 8 is now completed. Let's reflect:

What went well? _____
_____
_____

What did not go well? _____
_____
_____

Did I live in alignment with my goals? _____
_____
_____

If yes, what felt aligned? _____
    What can I do to strengthen this alignment in Week 9? _____
_____
_____

If no, what felt misaligned? _____
    What can I do differently in Week 9? _____
_____
_____

Answers easily flow to me

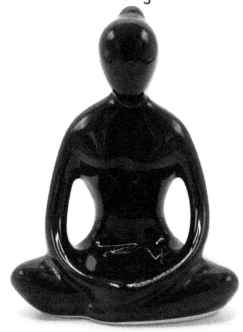

Week 9

Day 1   Date: _____

Today's Intention:

_____
_____
_____
_____

Today I am grateful for:

- _____
- _____
- _____

Which goal will I focus on today? _____

Day 2   Date: _____

Today's Intention:

_____
_____
_____
_____

Today I am grateful for:

- _____
- _____
- _____

Which goal will I focus on today? _____

Go to your 9th Self-Inquiry

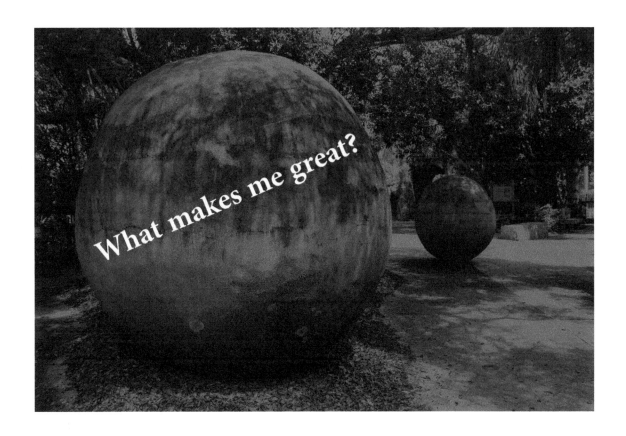

What makes me great?

_____
_____
_____
_____
_____
_____
_____
_____
_____
_____
_____
_____

What am I doing that is keeping me from realizing the full expression of my GREATNESS?

_____
_____
_____
_____
_____
_____
_____
_____
_____
_____

What would my life, my daily habits, my choices look like
if I fully connected with my **GREATNESS?**

Examples include:
- Daily, I would write for 15 minutes toward the completion of my screen play.
- Weekly, I would complete and update my To-Do or Action list for excellent time management.
- Every afternoon, I would engage in a 15-minute meditation practice.
- Every Sunday, I would write a special hand-written note showing appreciation for someone special.

Devise an ideal Day and Week plan and be specific of the **actions**
you would be taking:

Connecting my intentions to my goals	Daily I would:	Weekly I would:	Aligning my goals to my intentions

Finding my gifts   **Finding my Greatness**   Finding my Purpose

Day 3   Date_____

Today's Intention:

_____
_____
_____
_____

Today I am grateful for:

- _____
- _____
- _____

Which goal will I focus on today? _____

Day 4   Date: _____

Today's Intention:

_____
_____
_____
_____

Today I am grateful for:

- _____
- _____
- _____

Which goal will I focus on today? _____

Day 5   Date: _____

Today's Intention:

_____
_____
_____
_____

Today I am grateful for:
- _____
- _____
- _____

Which goal will I focus on today? _____

Day 6   Date: _____

Today's Intention:

_____
_____
_____
_____

Today I am grateful for:
- _____
- _____
- _____

Which goal will I focus on today? _____

Day 7   Date: _____

Today's Intention:

_____
_____
_____
_____

Today I am grateful for:
- _____
- _____
- _____

Which goal will I focus on today? _____

Go to Week 9's Let's Reflect

Week 9 is now completed. Let's reflect:

What went well? _____
_____
_____

What did not go well? _____
_____
_____

Did I live in alignment with my goals? _____
_____
_____

If yes, what felt aligned? _____
    What can I do to strengthen this alignment in Week 10? _____
_____
_____

If no, what felt misaligned? _____
    What can I do differently in Week 10? _____
_____
_____

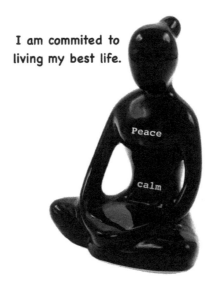

I am commited to
living my best life.

Peace

calm

Growing Stronger with Each Passing Day

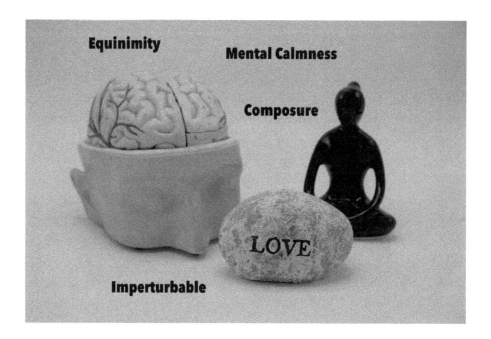

Just as I respect the Hebbian theory, I also deeply respect the
Pareto Principle (or the 80/20 rule).

Named after Vilfredo Pareto, an Italian economist, The Pareto Principle simply observes
that for many phenomena 80% of the results come from 20% of the effort.

Let's put this into everyday use:
80% of the time, we frequent only 20% of the restaurants and eateries nearby.
80% of the time, we wear only 20% of the clothes in our wardrobe.
80% of the referrals to your business come from 20% of our customers.
80% of the profits in our business come from 20% of our services and/or products.

The list goes on and on.

The 80/20 Rule can be a powerful formula for my life!

Pareto Meets Hebb
A Powerful Meeting

The brain, the nervous system, and the immune system are linked. They communicate
with and affect one another. Their synergy is staggering, and they are collectively coined
psychoneuroimmunology, or PNI for short. Prolonged stress weakens the immune
system, while prolonged states of calm strengthen it! We like prolonged states of calm.
Our brain likes it. Our nervous system likes it.

We can achieve it.
By ruthlessly taking inventory of your life and present circumstances and living according to your higher purpose, with both intention and integrity

&

pairing positive and healthy behaviors,
you are now set on a path of unstoppable success.
What's the one thing you can do that will make your day flow more easily?
What's the simplest action you can take that will promote your business?
What's the least you can do in a certain area in your life that will get you the most gain?
Here are some ideas to add healthy, immune
enhancing habits into your life.

Think in terms of Hebb and Pareto.

Is there a new habit I should incorporate in my life?

Is there anything presented in this list of recommended health habits that
if incorporated consistently in your life will add exponential value?

Hydrate; drink plenty of water	Increase plant-based food
Add dietary supplementation	Balance caloric intake
Get or improve restorative sleep	Establish a relaxing bedtime routine
Exercise (at least 150 minutes/week)	Practice yoga
Meditate	Manage your consumption of news
Listen to uplifting music	De-clutter and organize your living space
Listen to an uplifting or educational podcast	Go for a walk in or connect with nature
Volunteer	Read for fun
Enjoy a hobby	Write, draw, create

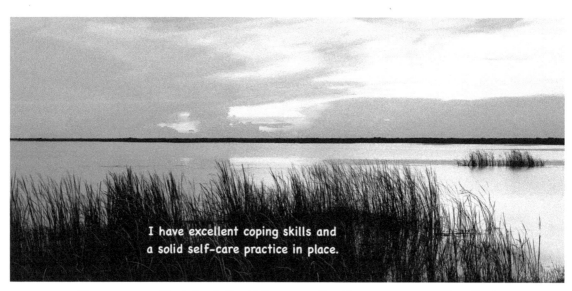

I have excellent coping skills and
a solid self-care practice in place.

Pareto & Hebb Meet <u>Csikszentmihalyi</u>

Remember our flow state positive psychologist?

By adding him to our powerful meeting, we will enter the zone or flow state much more often; meaning we will be operating from the space of highly focused mental productivity.

Use this opportunity to take inventory of your personal situation and how you spend your time.

> **Your time is the only thing that demonstrates what you care about.**
> -Tom Peters

Each and every time we give ourselves extra love, understand our patterns, enhance our self-awareness, we heal. Through healing, we give the best of ourselves to others. We bring amazing energy to any circumstance.
A healed mind is a peaceful mind.

What are some things you can be doing to maximize efficiency, productivity, happiness, peace, joy, etc.

_____
_____
_____
_____
_____
_____
_____
_____
_____
_____
_____
_____
_____
_____
_____
_____

What are some things you need to completely let go of because you're getting little if anything at all from that particular behavior, thought, action?

_____
_____
_____
_____
_____
_____
_____
_____
_____
_____
_____
_____
_____
_____
_____
_____
_____
_____
_____
_____

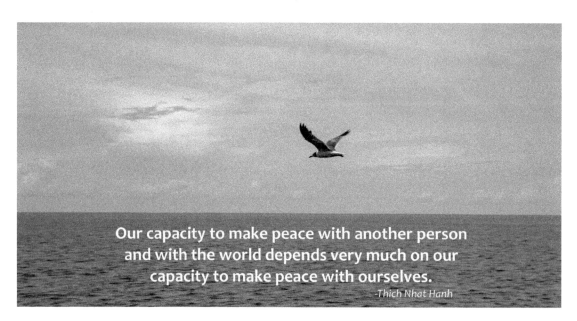

Our capacity to make peace with another person
and with the world depends very much on our
capacity to make peace with ourselves.
-Thich Nhat Hanh

Inhaling and Exhaling

Breathwork is an excellent practice to connect to the present moment.

As mentioned earlier, the practice of yoga has many benefits and at its root is proper breathing. Pranayama is the formal practice of controlling the breath, which is the source of prana (or life force). The importance of maintaining a steady, rhythmic breath is emphasized in yoga. The physical practice of yoga can be viewed as a moving meditation, incorporating the steadiness, sound and depth of the Ujjayi (or ocean) breath to help connect the mind and body, and achieve calmness.

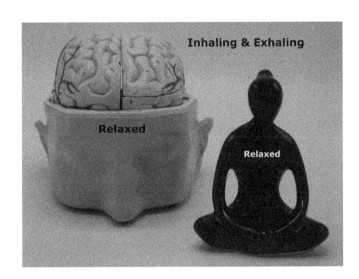

Here is a beginner's guide to accessing this breath:

- get into a comfortable seated position.
- breathe in through your nose and exhale through your mouth. Imagine you are fogging a mirror with your breath.
- when breathing, inhale to contract the diaphragm to create space for your lungs to expand, and when you exhale, relax the diaphragm and gently push the air from your lungs.
- Try to inhale and to exhale to a slow count of 4.

An extra benefit: practicing deep, proper breathing while connected with nature.

Ocean   Mountain   Lake   Forest   Park

Spend quality time outdoors.

Live in harmony with nature.

Week 10

Day 1   Date: _____

Today's Intention:

_____

_____

_____

_____

Today I am grateful for:

- _____
- _____
- _____

Which goal will I focus on today? _____

Day 2   Date: _____

Today's Intention:

_____

_____

_____

_____

Today I am grateful for:

- _____
- _____
- _____

Which goal will I focus on today? _____

Go to your 10th Self-Inquiry

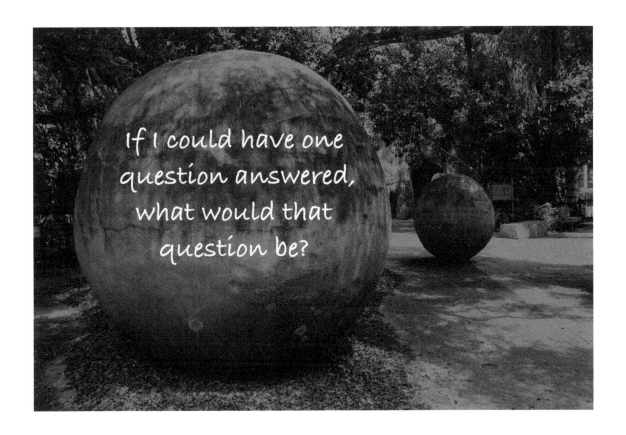

If I could have one question answered, what would that question be?

_____
_____
_____
_____
_____
_____

How would my life be different if I had the answer to this question?

_____
_____
_____
_____

What would I do and how would I feel if the answer to this question never comes or if it will be a long while?

_____
_____
_____
_____
_____
_____

Day 3   Date_____

Today's Intention:

_____
_____
_____
_____

Today I am grateful for:
- _____
- _____
- _____

Which goal will I focus on today? _____

Day 4   Date: _____

Today's Intention:

_____
_____
_____
_____

Today I am grateful for:
- _____
- _____
- _____

Which goal will I focus on today? _____

Day 5   Date: _____

Today's Intention:

_____
_____
_____
_____

Today I am grateful for:

- _____
- _____
- _____

Which goal will I focus on today? _____

Day 6   Date: _____

Today's Intention:

_____
_____
_____
_____

Today I am grateful for:

- _____
- _____
- _____

Which goal will I focus on today? _____

Day 7   Date: _____

Today's Intention:

_____
_____
_____
_____

Today I am grateful for:

- _____
- _____
- _____

Which goal will I focus on today? _____

Go to Week 10's Let's Reflect

Week 10 is now completed. Let's reflect:

What went well? _____
_____
_____

What did not go well? _____
_____
_____

Did I live in alignment with my goals? _____
_____
_____

If yes, what felt aligned? _____
    What can I do to strengthen this alignment in the upcoming weeks? _____
_____
_____

If no, what felt misaligned? _____
    What can I do differently in the upcoming weeks? _____
_____
_____

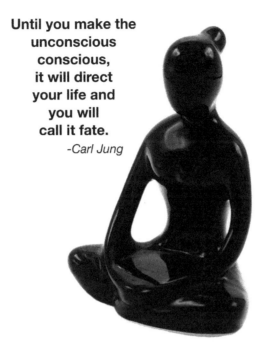

**Until you make the
unconscious
conscious,
it will direct
your life and
you will
call it fate.**
-Carl Jung

Congratulations

You now know yourself better than you did at the start of this self-inquiry journey.
This is only the beginning.
Each day we begin anew.
We can never run out of self-growth opportunities.

Re-visit any or all of these questions at a later time.
Different feelings and/or thoughts will emerge.

Just as we cannot enter the same river twice, we are
changed by experience, growth, & connection.

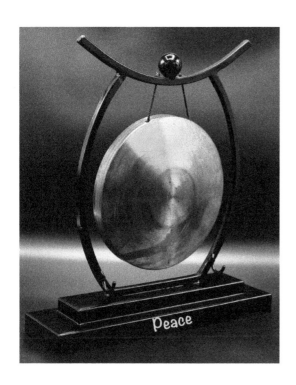

Remember, we can

Re-start
Re-do
Re-focus
RENEW

as often as we need to!

What is success?
It is being able to go to bed each night
with your soul at peace.
-Paulo Coelho

And tomorrow we begin again!

INSPIRATIONS

Notes /Thoughts/ Ideas

I have been inspired by the following book(s): _____
_____
_____
_____

I have been inspired by the following movie(s): _____
_____
_____
_____

I have been inspired by the following song(s): _____
_____
_____
_____
_____
_____
_____
_____
_____
_____
_____
_____
_____
_____
_____
_____
_____
_____
_____
_____

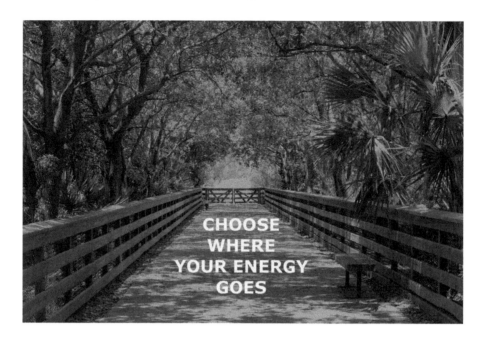

CHOOSE
WHERE
YOUR ENERGY
GOES

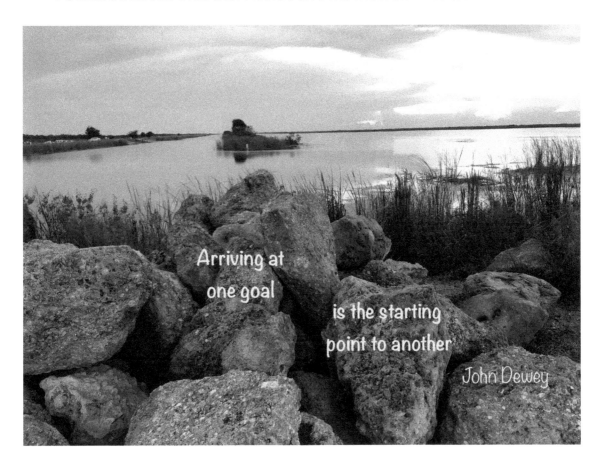

Arriving at
one goal
is the starting
point to another
John Dewey

A journey of 1000 miles begins with a single step.

Next Step: Keep this journal in a safe place and in the weeks and months to come, I invite you to review it; several times at different time frames.

Powerful insights will occur.

It will be interesting to see how your life, your goals, your choices,
your habits have changed.

Progress is measured by how far we've come, not how far we still need to go.

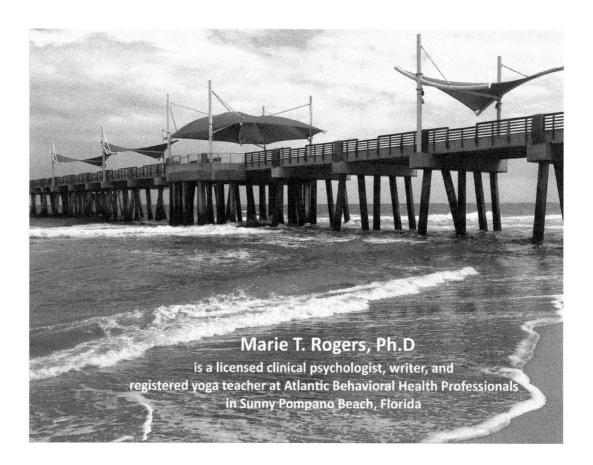

Marie T. Rogers, Ph.D
is a licensed clinical psychologist, writer, and
registered yoga teacher at Atlantic Behavioral Health Professionals
in Sunny Pompano Beach, Florida

Let's connect:

 Marie Therese Rogers
Atlantic Behavioral Health Professionals

 Marie T. Rogers, Ph.D.

 mariethereserogers

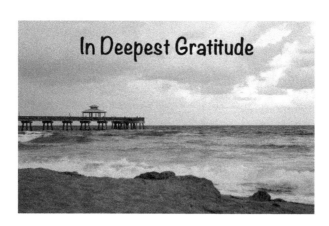

In Deepest Gratitude

CPSIA information can be obtained
at www.ICGtesting.com
Printed in the USA
BVHW021346050821
613728BV00010B/405